RENAL DIET COOKBOOK FOR SENIORS

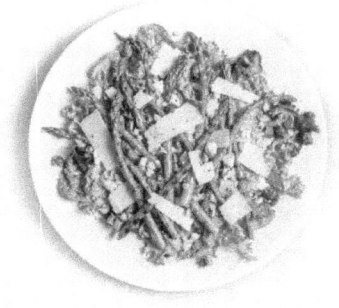

DR. JESSICA SMITH

Copyright © 2024 by DR. JESSICA SMITH

All rights reserved.

No part of this book may be reproduced, stored in a retrieval system, or transmitted, in any form or by any means, electronic, mechanical, photocopying, recording, or otherwise, without prior written permission from the publisher, except for brief quotations embodied in critical articles or reviews.

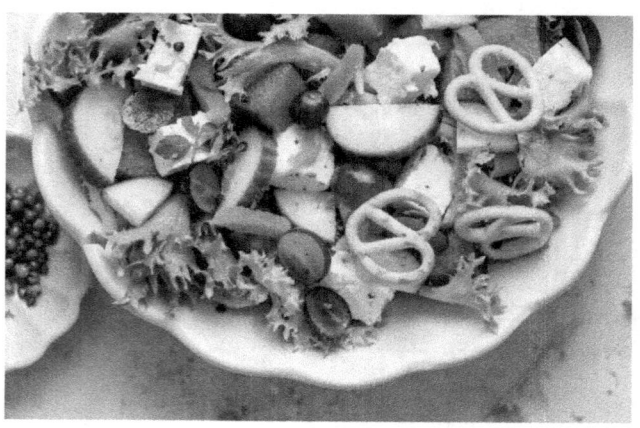

TABLE OF CONTENTS

CHAPTER ONE 7

How to Use this Cookbook 7

Understanding Renal Diet for Seniors 8

Benefits of Renal Diet for Seniors 10

Guidelines for Renal Diet for Seniors 12

CHAPTER TWO 15

Renal Diet Breakfast Recipes for Seniors 15

1: Veggie Omelette 15

2: Overnight Oats with Berries 16

3: Greek Yogurt Parfait 18

4: Quinoa Breakfast Bowl 19

5: Sweet Potato Breakfast Hash 21

6: Cottage Cheese with Fruit 22

7: Spinach and Mushroom Egg Muffins. 24

8: Apple Cinnamon Quinoa Porridge 25

9: Avocado Toast with Poached Egg 27

10: Chia Seed Pudding 29

Renal Diet Lunch Recipes for Seniors ... 30

1: Grilled Salmon with Lemon-Dill Sauce 30

2: Quinoa and Vegetable Stir-Fry 32

3: Lentil and Vegetable Soup 34

4: Turkey and Avocado Wrap 36

5: Quinoa Salad with Chickpeas and Vegetables 37

6: Tuna Salad Lettuce Wraps 39

7: Chicken and Vegetable Stir-Fry 41

8: Egg Salad Lettuce Wraps 43

9: Vegetable and Bean Quinoa Salad 44

10: Turkey and Vegetable Skewers 46

Renal Diet Dinner Recipes for Seniors ... 47

1: Baked Lemon Herb Chicken 47

2: Salmon and Asparagus Foil Packets ... 49

3: Turkey and Vegetable Stir-Fry 51

4: Lentil and Vegetable Curry 53

5: Grilled Lemon Garlic Shrimp Skewers 55

6: Baked Herb-Crusted Cod 57

7: Vegetable and Bean Chili 59

8: Lemon Herb Baked Chicken Thighs .. 61

9: Baked Salmon with Roasted Vegetables 63

10: Turkey and Vegetable Skillet............65

Renal Diet Snacks Recipes for Seniors ..66

1: Greek Yogurt and Berry Parfait..........66

2: Veggie Sticks with Hummus...............68

3: Cottage Cheese and Fruit Bowl..........69

4: Avocado and Tomato Toast 70

5: Egg Salad Cucumber Bites 72

6: Almond Butter Apple Slices 73

7: Tuna and Cucumber Roll-Ups 75

8: Rice Cake with Avocado and Tomato 76

9: Hummus-Stuffed Mini Bell Peppers ..78

10: Cottage Cheese and Tomato Slices ..79

CONCLUSION...81

CHAPTER ONE

How to Use this Cookbook

Understand the Basics: Begin by familiarizing yourself with the principles of a renal diet. This typically involves limiting certain nutrients like sodium, potassium, and phosphorus while ensuring adequate protein intake.

Read the Introduction: Start by reading the introduction of the cookbook. This section often includes valuable information about renal diet guidelines, ingredient substitutions, and cooking tips.

Review the Recipes: Take some time to browse through the recipes in the cookbook.

Pay attention to the ingredients and nutritional information provided with each recipe.

Plan Your Meals: Plan your meals for the week based on the recipes you find in the cookbook. Consider incorporating a variety of dishes to ensure a balanced diet.

Make a Shopping List: Once you've chosen your recipes, make a shopping list of the ingredients you'll need.

This will help you stay organized and ensure you have everything on hand when it's time to cook.

Follow the Recipes Carefully: When cooking, follow the recipes in the cookbook carefully, paying attention to portion sizes and cooking instructions. This will help you achieve the desired nutritional balance.

Adjust for Personal Preferences: Feel free to adjust the recipes to suit your personal preferences and dietary needs. You can often swap ingredients or adjust seasoning to taste.

Monitor Portion Sizes: Keep track of portion sizes to ensure you're not consuming too much of any particular nutrient. This is especially important when it comes to ingredients like salt, potassium, and phosphorus.

Enjoy Your Meals: Finally, sit down and enjoy the delicious and nutritious meals you've prepared using the renal diet cookbook. Eating well is an important part of maintaining overall health and well-being.

Understanding Renal Diet for Seniors

Understanding the renal diet for seniors is crucial for maintaining optimal health, particularly for those with kidney issues or related conditions. This specialized diet focuses on managing the intake of certain nutrients to alleviate stress on the kidneys and prevent complications.

Here are key aspects to comprehend:

Firstly, the renal diet emphasizes controlling the consumption of sodium, potassium, and phosphorus.

Excessive intake of these minerals can strain the kidneys, leading to fluid retention, electrolyte imbalances, and other complications. Seniors need to be mindful of hidden sources of these minerals in processed and packaged foods.

Secondly, protein intake is moderated in the renal diet. While protein is essential for muscle strength and overall health, too much can burden the kidneys. Seniors are advised to choose high-quality protein sources and monitor portion sizes.

Thirdly, fluid intake is regulated to prevent fluid overload, which can exacerbate kidney issues and increase blood pressure. Seniors should be mindful of their thirst cues and limit fluids accordingly, especially if advised by a healthcare professional.

Finally, individualized dietary plans are essential. Seniors may have varying degrees of kidney function and medical conditions, so consulting with a healthcare provider or dietitian is crucial to tailor the renal diet to individual needs and preferences.

Benefits of Renal Diet for Seniors

The benefits of a renal diet for seniors are numerous, particularly for those managing kidney disease or related conditions.

Here are some key advantages:

Kidney Health Maintenance: A renal diet helps seniors manage kidney function by regulating the intake of sodium, potassium, phosphorus, and protein. By controlling these nutrients, the diet reduces strain on the kidneys and helps prevent further damage.

Blood Pressure Control: Many seniors with kidney issues also struggle with high blood pressure. The renal diet, which typically limits sodium intake, can help lower blood pressure levels, reducing the risk of heart disease and stroke.

Fluid Balance: Seniors on a renal diet learn to manage their fluid intake, preventing fluid overload that can exacerbate kidney problems. Proper fluid balance is crucial for maintaining healthy blood pressure and avoiding complications like edema and shortness of breath.

Nutritional Support: Despite restrictions on certain nutrients, a well-planned renal diet ensures seniors receive adequate nutrition. High-quality protein sources, essential vitamins, and minerals are emphasized, supporting overall health and well-being.

Symptom Management: Following a renal diet can alleviate symptoms associated with kidney disease, such as fatigue, nausea, and swelling. By optimizing nutrition and minimizing stress on the kidneys, seniors may experience improved energy levels and overall quality of life.

Reduced Risk of Complications: By adhering to a renal diet, seniors can reduce the risk of complications associated with kidney disease, such as electrolyte imbalances, bone health issues, and cardiovascular problems.

Guidelines for Renal Diet for Seniors

Adhering to specific guidelines is essential for seniors following a renal diet, designed to support kidney health and overall well-being.

Here are key principles to consider:

Limit Sodium Intake: Seniors should aim to reduce their sodium intake to help control blood pressure and fluid retention.

This involves avoiding processed and high-sodium foods, opting for fresh ingredients, and using herbs and spices for flavor instead of salt.

Monitor Potassium Levels: Seniors with kidney issues need to manage their potassium intake to prevent heart rhythm disturbances. Foods high in potassium, such as bananas, oranges, and tomatoes, should be consumed in moderation or under guidance from a healthcare provider.

Control Phosphorus Intake: Phosphorus levels need to be regulated to prevent bone and heart complications. Seniors should limit phosphorus-rich foods like dairy products, nuts, and whole grains and choose low-phosphorus alternatives when possible.

Moderate Protein Consumption: While protein is essential, seniors on a renal diet should moderate their intake to reduce stress on the kidneys. Opt for high-quality protein sources like lean meats, fish, eggs, and legumes, and monitor portion sizes accordingly.

Manage Fluid Intake: Seniors should monitor their fluid intake to avoid fluid overload, which can strain the kidneys and lead to complications. It's important to balance fluid intake with thirst cues and recommendations from healthcare providers.

Individualized Approach: Since kidney function can vary among seniors, it's crucial to tailor the renal diet to individual needs and medical conditions.

Consulting with a healthcare provider or dietitian can help seniors develop a personalized dietary plan that supports their kidney health and overall well-being.

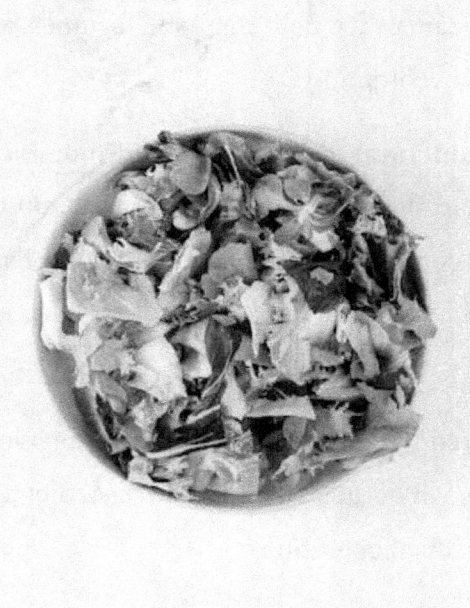

CHAPTER TWO

Renal Diet Breakfast Recipes for Seniors

1: Veggie Omelette

Ingredients:

- 2 eggs
- 1/4 cup diced bell peppers
- 1/4 cup diced onions
- 1/4 cup diced tomatoes
- 1/4 cup chopped spinach
- Salt and pepper to taste
- 1 teaspoon olive oil

Instructions:

- Heat olive oil in a non-stick skillet over medium heat.
- In a bowl, beat the eggs with salt and pepper.
- Pour the beaten eggs into the skillet and swirl to coat the bottom evenly.
- Cook for 2-3 minutes until the edges start to set.

- Sprinkle the diced bell peppers, onions, tomatoes, and spinach evenly over one half of the omelette.
- Gently fold the other half of the omelette over the vegetables.
- Cook for another 2-3 minutes until the vegetables are tender and the eggs are cooked through.
- Slide the omelette onto a plate and serve hot.

Health Benefits:

- High in protein from eggs, which is important for muscle strength.
- Packed with vitamins and minerals from vegetables, supporting overall health.
- Low in sodium, potassium, and phosphorus, making it kidney-friendly.

Preparation Time: 10 minutes

2: Overnight Oats with Berries

Ingredients:

- 1/2 cup rolled oats
- 1/2 cup unsweetened almond milk

- 1/4 cup mixed berries (such as strawberries, blueberries, raspberries)
- 1 tablespoon chopped almonds
- 1 teaspoon honey or maple syrup (optional)
- 1/4 teaspoon vanilla extract (optional)

Instructions:

- In a mason jar or container, combine rolled oats and almond milk.
- Add the mixed berries, chopped almonds, honey or maple syrup (if using), and vanilla extract (if using).
- Stir well to combine all ingredients.
- Cover the jar with a lid and refrigerate overnight.
- In the morning, give the oats a good stir and add a splash of almond milk if desired.
- Enjoy cold or heat in the microwave for 1-2 minutes before serving.

Health Benefits:

- Oats are high in fiber, aiding digestion and promoting heart health.

- Berries are rich in antioxidants, reducing inflammation and supporting immune function.
- Almonds provide healthy fats and protein, keeping you full and satisfied.
- Low in sodium, potassium, and phosphorus, suitable for a renal diet.

Preparation Time: 5 minutes (plus overnight refrigeration)

3: Greek Yogurt Parfait

Ingredients:

- 1/2 cup low-fat Greek yogurt
- 1/4 cup fresh mixed berries (such as strawberries, blueberries, raspberries)
- 1 tablespoon chopped walnuts
- 1 teaspoon honey (optional)
- 1/4 teaspoon cinnamon (optional)

Instructions:

- In a serving bowl or glass, layer the Greek yogurt, mixed berries, and chopped walnuts.
- Drizzle honey over the top if desired, and sprinkle with cinnamon.

- Repeat the layering process until all ingredients are used.
- Serve immediately.

Health Benefits:

- Greek yogurt is high in protein and calcium, supporting bone health and muscle function.
- Berries provide antioxidants and fiber, promoting heart health and digestion.
- Walnuts offer healthy fats and omega-3 fatty acids, reducing inflammation and supporting brain health.
- Low in sodium, potassium, and phosphorus, suitable for a renal diet.

Preparation Time: 5 minutes

4: Quinoa Breakfast Bowl

Ingredients:

- 1/2 cup cooked quinoa
- 1/4 cup sliced banana
- 1 tablespoon chopped almonds
- 1 tablespoon dried cranberries
- 1 teaspoon honey or maple syrup (optional)

- 1/4 teaspoon cinnamon (optional)

Instructions:

- In a bowl, combine the cooked quinoa, sliced banana, chopped almonds, and dried cranberries.
- Drizzle honey or maple syrup over the top if desired, and sprinkle with cinnamon.
- Stir well to combine all ingredients.
- Serve immediately.

Health Benefits:

- Quinoa is a complete protein, providing all essential amino acids and supporting muscle repair and growth.
- Bananas are rich in potassium and fiber, promoting heart health and digestion.
- Almonds offer healthy fats and protein, keeping you full and satisfied.
- Cranberries provide antioxidants and may help prevent urinary tract infections.
- Low in sodium, suitable for a renal diet.

Preparation Time: 10 minutes (if quinoa is already cooked)

5: Sweet Potato Breakfast Hash

Ingredients:

- 1 small sweet potato, peeled and diced
- 1/4 cup diced bell peppers
- 1/4 cup diced onions
- 1/4 cup diced zucchini
- 1 tablespoon olive oil
- Salt and pepper to taste
- 2 eggs (optional)

Instructions:

- Heat olive oil in a skillet over medium heat.
- Add the diced sweet potato to the skillet and cook for 5-7 minutes until lightly browned and tender.
- Add the diced bell peppers, onions, and zucchini to the skillet and cook for an additional 3-4 minutes until vegetables are tender.
- Season with salt and pepper to taste.
- If desired, create wells in the hash and crack eggs into each well.
- Cover the skillet and cook for 3-5 minutes until eggs are cooked to your preference.

- Serve hot.

Health Benefits:

- Sweet potatoes are rich in vitamins A and C, fiber, and antioxidants, supporting immune function and digestive health.
- Bell peppers and zucchini add additional vitamins and minerals while being low in potassium and phosphorus.
- Eggs provide high-quality protein and essential nutrients, aiding in muscle strength and overall health.
- Low in sodium, suitable for a renal diet.

Preparation Time: 15 minutes

6: Cottage Cheese with Fruit

Ingredients:

- 1/2 cup low-fat cottage cheese
- 1/4 cup diced pineapple
- 1/4 cup diced mango
- 1 tablespoon shredded coconut
- 1 tablespoon chopped walnuts (optional)

- 1 teaspoon honey or maple syrup (optional)

Instructions:

- In a bowl, combine the low-fat cottage cheese, diced pineapple, diced mango, shredded coconut, and chopped walnuts (if using).
- Drizzle honey or maple syrup over the top if desired.
- Stir well to combine all ingredients.
- Serve immediately.

Health Benefits:

- Cottage cheese is a good source of protein and calcium, supporting bone health and muscle function.
- Pineapple and mango provide vitamins, minerals, and antioxidants, promoting immune function and digestive health.
- Walnuts offer healthy fats and omega-3 fatty acids, reducing inflammation and supporting heart health.
- Low in sodium and phosphorus, suitable for a renal diet.

Preparation Time: 5 minutes

7: Spinach and Mushroom Egg Muffins

Ingredients:

- 4 large eggs
- 1 cup chopped spinach
- 1/2 cup diced mushrooms
- 1/4 cup diced onions
- Salt and pepper to taste
- Cooking spray or olive oil

Instructions:

- Preheat the oven to 350°F (175°C). Grease a muffin tin with cooking spray or olive oil.
- In a bowl, whisk together the eggs, salt, and pepper.
- Stir in the chopped spinach, diced mushrooms, and diced onions until well combined.
- Pour the egg mixture evenly into the prepared muffin tin, filling each cup about 3/4 full.
- Bake in the preheated oven for 20-25 minutes, or until the egg muffins are set and lightly golden on top.
- Allow the egg muffins to cool slightly before removing them from the muffin tin.

- Serve warm or store in an airtight container in the refrigerator for up to 3 days.

Health Benefits:

- Eggs are a good source of protein and essential nutrients, supporting muscle strength and overall health.
- Spinach is rich in vitamins, minerals, and antioxidants, promoting heart health and immune function.
- Mushrooms and onions add flavor and additional vitamins while being low in potassium and phosphorus.
- Low in sodium, suitable for a renal diet.

Preparation Time: 30 minutes

8: Apple Cinnamon Quinoa Porridge

Ingredients:

- 1/2 cup cooked quinoa
- 1/2 cup unsweetened almond milk
- 1 small apple, peeled and diced
- 1 tablespoon chopped walnuts

- 1 tablespoon raisins
- 1/2 teaspoon cinnamon
- 1 teaspoon honey or maple syrup (optional)

Instructions:

- In a small saucepan, combine the cooked quinoa, almond milk, diced apple, chopped walnuts, raisins, and cinnamon.
- Cook over medium heat, stirring occasionally, until the mixture is heated through and the apple is tender, about 5-7 minutes.
- If desired, drizzle honey or maple syrup over the top for added sweetness.
- Serve warm.

Health Benefits:

- Quinoa provides protein, fiber, and essential nutrients, supporting muscle repair and digestive health.
- Apples are rich in fiber and antioxidants, promoting heart health and digestion.

- Walnuts offer healthy fats and omega-3 fatty acids, reducing inflammation and supporting brain health.
- Low in sodium, suitable for a renal diet.

Preparation Time: 10 minutes

9: Avocado Toast with Poached Egg

Ingredients:

- 1 slice whole grain bread
- 1/2 ripe avocado
- 1 egg
- Salt and pepper to taste
- Optional toppings: cherry tomatoes, sliced cucumber, microgreens

Instructions:

- Toast the whole grain bread until golden brown.
- While the bread is toasting, mash the ripe avocado in a small bowl and season with salt and pepper to taste.
- Poach the egg: Bring a small pot of water to a gentle simmer. Crack the egg into a small bowl or ramekin. Create a gentle whirlpool in the simmering water with a spoon and carefully slide the egg into the

center. Cook for 3-4 minutes, until the egg whites are set but the yolk is still runny.
- Remove the poached egg with a slotted spoon and drain on a paper towel.
- Spread the mashed avocado evenly on the toasted bread.
- Top with the poached egg and optional toppings, if desired.
- Serve immediately.

Health Benefits:

- Whole grain bread provides fiber and complex carbohydrates, promoting digestive health and stable blood sugar levels.
- Avocado is rich in healthy fats, vitamins, and minerals, supporting heart health and brain function.
- Eggs offer high-quality protein and essential nutrients, aiding in muscle repair and overall health.
- Low in sodium and potassium, suitable for a renal diet.

Preparation Time: 10 minutes

10: Chia Seed Pudding

Ingredients:

- 2 tablespoons chia seeds
- 1/2 cup unsweetened almond milk
- 1/4 teaspoon vanilla extract
- 1 teaspoon honey or maple syrup (optional)
- Fresh fruit for topping (such as berries or sliced banana)

Instructions:

- In a small bowl or jar, combine the chia seeds, almond milk, vanilla extract, and honey or maple syrup (if using).
- Stir well to combine all ingredients.
- Cover and refrigerate for at least 2 hours, or preferably overnight, to allow the chia seeds to absorb the liquid and thicken.
- Stir the chia seed pudding before serving to ensure a creamy consistency.
- Top with fresh fruit before serving.

Health Benefits:

- Chia seeds are rich in fiber, protein, and omega-3 fatty acids, promoting digestive health, satiety, and heart health.
- Almond milk is low in calories and contains no cholesterol or saturated fat, making it a heart-healthy alternative to dairy milk.
- Fresh fruit provides vitamins, minerals, and antioxidants, supporting immune function and overall health.
- Low in sodium and potassium, suitable for a renal diet.

Preparation Time: 5 minutes (plus chilling time)

Renal Diet Lunch Recipes for Seniors

1: Grilled Salmon with Lemon-Dill Sauce

Ingredients:

- 1 salmon fillet (4-6 ounces)
- 1 tablespoon olive oil
- Salt and pepper to taste
- 1 lemon

- 1 tablespoon chopped fresh dill
- 1 tablespoon Greek yogurt (optional)

Instructions:

- Preheat the grill to medium-high heat.
- Brush the salmon fillet with olive oil and season with salt and pepper.
- Slice half of the lemon into thin rounds and reserve the other half for squeezing juice.
- Grill the salmon fillet for 4-5 minutes per side, or until cooked through and flaky.
- Meanwhile, prepare the lemon-dill sauce by mixing the juice from the reserved lemon half with chopped fresh dill and Greek yogurt (if using).
- Serve the grilled salmon with lemon-dill sauce on top and garnish with lemon rounds.
- Enjoy with a side of steamed vegetables or a green salad.

Health Benefits:

- Salmon is rich in omega-3 fatty acids, which can reduce inflammation and support heart health.

- Lemon provides vitamin C and antioxidants, boosting immune function and aiding in digestion.
- Dill is a good source of vitamins A and C, promoting bone health and supporting immune function.
- Greek yogurt adds creaminess and protein to the sauce, supporting muscle strength.

Preparation Time: 15 minutes

2: Quinoa and Vegetable Stir-Fry

Ingredients:

- 1/2 cup cooked quinoa
- 1 cup mixed vegetables (such as bell peppers, broccoli, carrots, snap peas)
- 2 tablespoons low-sodium soy sauce
- 1 tablespoon olive oil
- 2 cloves garlic, minced
- 1 teaspoon grated ginger
- Salt and pepper to taste
- Optional: cooked chicken, tofu, or shrimp for protein

Instructions:

- Heat olive oil in a large skillet or wok over medium heat.
- Add minced garlic and grated ginger to the skillet and cook for 1-2 minutes until fragrant.
- Add mixed vegetables to the skillet and stir-fry for 5-7 minutes until tender-crisp.
- Stir in cooked quinoa and optional protein (if using) until heated through.
- Drizzle low-sodium soy sauce over the quinoa and vegetable mixture, and toss to coat evenly.
- Season with salt and pepper to taste.
- Serve hot.

Health Benefits:

- Quinoa is a complete protein and rich in fiber, aiding in muscle repair and promoting digestive health.
- Mixed vegetables provide vitamins, minerals, and antioxidants, supporting immune function and overall health.

- Garlic and ginger have anti-inflammatory properties and may help lower blood pressure and cholesterol levels.
- Low-sodium soy sauce adds flavor without increasing sodium intake.

Preparation Time: 20 minutes

3: Lentil and Vegetable Soup

Ingredients:

- 1/2 cup dried green lentils, rinsed
- 4 cups low-sodium vegetable broth
- 1 carrot, diced
- 1 celery stalk, diced
- 1/2 onion, diced
- 1 clove garlic, minced
- 1 teaspoon olive oil
- 1/2 teaspoon dried thyme
- Salt and pepper to taste
- Fresh parsley for garnish

Instructions:

- Heat olive oil in a large pot over medium heat.
- Add diced onion, carrot, and celery to the pot and sauté for 5-7 minutes until softened.
- Add minced garlic and dried thyme to the pot and cook for an additional 1-2 minutes until fragrant.
- Pour in low-sodium vegetable broth and add rinsed lentils to the pot.
- Bring the soup to a boil, then reduce heat to low and simmer for 20-25 minutes until lentils are tender.
- Season with salt and pepper to taste.
- Ladle the soup into bowls and garnish with fresh parsley before serving.

Health Benefits:

- Lentils are high in protein and fiber, promoting satiety and supporting digestive health.
- Vegetables add vitamins, minerals, and antioxidants, boosting immune function and overall health.
- Olive oil provides healthy fats and may help reduce inflammation and improve heart health.

- Low-sodium vegetable broth ensures the soup is kidney-friendly.

Preparation Time: 30 minutes

4: Turkey and Avocado Wrap

Ingredients:

- 1 whole wheat tortilla
- 2 slices roasted turkey breast
- 1/4 avocado, sliced
- 1/4 cup shredded lettuce
- 2 slices tomato
- 1 tablespoon hummus
- Salt and pepper to taste

Instructions:

- Lay the whole wheat tortilla flat on a clean surface.
- Spread hummus evenly over the tortilla.
- Layer roasted turkey breast, sliced avocado, shredded lettuce, and tomato slices on top of the hummus.
- Season with salt and pepper to taste.
- Roll up the tortilla tightly into a wrap.

- Cut the wrap in half diagonally and secure with toothpicks if desired.
- Serve immediately, or wrap in parchment paper for later.

Health Benefits:

- Whole wheat tortillas provide fiber and complex carbohydrates, promoting digestive health and stable blood sugar levels.
- Turkey breast is a lean source of protein, supporting muscle strength and repair.
- Avocado adds healthy fats, vitamins, and minerals, supporting heart health and brain function.
- Hummus provides additional protein and fiber, aiding in satiety and digestive health.

Preparation Time: 10 minutes

5: Quinoa Salad with Chickpeas and Vegetables

Ingredients:

- 1/2 cup cooked quinoa

- 1/2 cup cooked chickpeas (canned, drained, and rinsed)
- 1/2 cup diced cucumber
- 1/2 cup diced bell peppers (any color)
- 1/4 cup diced red onion
- 2 tablespoons chopped fresh parsley
- Juice of 1 lemon
- 1 tablespoon olive oil
- Salt and pepper to taste

Instructions:

- In a large bowl, combine the cooked quinoa, chickpeas, diced cucumber, diced bell peppers, diced red onion, and chopped fresh parsley.
- Drizzle lemon juice and olive oil over the salad, and toss until well combined.
- Season with salt and pepper to taste.
- Serve immediately, or refrigerate for later.

Health Benefits:

- Quinoa is a complete protein and rich in fiber, promoting muscle repair and digestive health.

- Chickpeas provide protein, fiber, and essential nutrients, aiding in satiety and overall health.
- Vegetables add vitamins, minerals, and antioxidants, supporting immune function and heart health.
- Lemon juice and olive oil provide flavor and healthy fats, promoting heart health and reducing inflammation.

Preparation Time: 15 minutes

6: Tuna Salad Lettuce Wraps

Ingredients:

- 1 can (5 ounces) tuna, drained
- 2 tablespoons Greek yogurt
- 1 tablespoon lemon juice
- 1 tablespoon chopped fresh dill
- 1/4 cup diced cucumber
- 1/4 cup diced bell peppers (any color)
- Salt and pepper to taste
- 4 large lettuce leaves (such as butter lettuce or romaine)

Instructions:

- In a mixing bowl, combine the drained tuna, Greek yogurt, lemon juice, chopped fresh dill, diced cucumber, and diced bell peppers.
- Stir until all ingredients are well combined.
- Season with salt and pepper to taste.
- Divide the tuna salad mixture evenly among the large lettuce leaves.
- Roll up the lettuce leaves to form wraps.
- Serve immediately.

Health Benefits:

- Tuna is a lean source of protein and omega-3 fatty acids, supporting muscle strength and heart health.
- Greek yogurt adds creaminess and protein to the salad, aiding in muscle repair and promoting satiety.
- Vegetables provide vitamins, minerals, and antioxidants, boosting immune function and overall health.
- Lettuce leaves serve as a low-carb alternative to traditional wraps, reducing calorie and carbohydrate intake.

Preparation Time: 10 minutes

7: Chicken and Vegetable Stir-Fry

Ingredients:

- 4 ounces boneless, skinless chicken breast, sliced
- 1 cup mixed vegetables (such as broccoli, bell peppers, snap peas)
- 1 tablespoon low-sodium soy sauce
- 1 tablespoon olive oil
- 1 clove garlic, minced
- 1 teaspoon grated ginger
- Salt and pepper to taste
- Cooked brown rice or quinoa for serving (optional)

Instructions:

- Heat olive oil in a large skillet or wok over medium-high heat.
- Add sliced chicken breast to the skillet and cook for 4-5 minutes until browned and cooked through.
- Remove the cooked chicken from the skillet and set aside.

- In the same skillet, add minced garlic and grated ginger, and cook for 1-2 minutes until fragrant.
- Add mixed vegetables to the skillet and stir-fry for 5-7 minutes until tender-crisp.
- Return the cooked chicken to the skillet and stir to combine with the vegetables.
- Drizzle low-sodium soy sauce over the chicken and vegetables, and toss to coat evenly.
- Season with salt and pepper to taste.
- Serve hot over cooked brown rice or quinoa, if desired.

Health Benefits:

- Chicken breast is a lean source of protein, supporting muscle strength and repair.
- Mixed vegetables provide vitamins, minerals, and antioxidants, supporting immune function and overall health.
- Garlic and ginger have anti-inflammatory properties and may help lower blood pressure and cholesterol levels.

- Low-sodium soy sauce adds flavor without increasing sodium intake.

Preparation Time: 20 minutes

8: Egg Salad Lettuce Wraps

Ingredients:

- 4 hard-boiled eggs, chopped
- 2 tablespoons Greek yogurt
- 1 tablespoon Dijon mustard
- 1 tablespoon chopped fresh dill or chives
- Salt and pepper to taste
- 4 large lettuce leaves (such as butter lettuce or romaine)

Instructions:

- In a mixing bowl, combine the chopped hard-boiled eggs, Greek yogurt, Dijon mustard, chopped fresh dill or chives, salt, and pepper.
- Stir until all ingredients are well combined.
- Divide the egg salad mixture evenly among the large lettuce leaves.
- Roll up the lettuce leaves to form wraps.

- Serve immediately.

Health Benefits:

- Eggs provide high-quality protein and essential nutrients, supporting muscle strength and overall health.
- Greek yogurt adds creaminess and protein to the salad, aiding in muscle repair and promoting satiety.
- Dijon mustard and fresh herbs add flavor without extra calories or sodium.
- Lettuce leaves serve as a low-carb alternative to traditional wraps, reducing calorie and carbohydrate intake.

Preparation Time: 10 minutes

9: Vegetable and Bean Quinoa Salad

Ingredients:

- 1/2 cup cooked quinoa
- 1/2 cup cooked black beans (canned, drained, and rinsed)
- 1/2 cup diced tomatoes
- 1/4 cup diced bell peppers (any color)

- 1/4 cup diced red onion
- 2 tablespoons chopped fresh cilantro
- Juice of 1 lime
- 1 tablespoon olive oil
- Salt and pepper to taste

Instructions:

- In a large bowl, combine the cooked quinoa, black beans, diced tomatoes, diced bell peppers, diced red onion, and chopped fresh cilantro.
- Drizzle lime juice and olive oil over the salad, and toss until well combined.
- Season with salt and pepper to taste.
- Serve immediately, or refrigerate for later.

Health Benefits:

- Quinoa is a complete protein and rich in fiber, promoting muscle repair and digestive health.
- Black beans provide protein, fiber, and essential nutrients, aiding in satiety and overall health.
- Vegetables add vitamins, minerals, and antioxidants, supporting immune function and heart health.

- Lime juice and olive oil provide flavor and healthy fats, promoting heart health and reducing inflammation.

Preparation Time: 15 minutes

10: Turkey and Vegetable Skewers

Ingredients:

- 4 ounces turkey breast, cut into cubes
- 1/2 zucchini, sliced
- 1/2 yellow bell pepper, cut into chunks
- 1/2 red onion, cut into chunks
- 1 tablespoon olive oil
- 1 teaspoon dried Italian seasoning
- Salt and pepper to taste

Instructions:

- Preheat the grill or grill pan to medium-high heat.
- Thread the turkey cubes, zucchini slices, yellow bell pepper chunks, and red onion chunks onto skewers, alternating between ingredients.
- Brush the skewers with olive oil and sprinkle with dried Italian seasoning, salt, and pepper.

- Grill the skewers for 8-10 minutes, turning occasionally, until the turkey is cooked through and the vegetables are tender.
- Remove the skewers from the grill and serve hot.

Health Benefits:

- Turkey breast is a lean source of protein, supporting muscle strength and repair.
- Zucchini, bell pepper, and red onion provide vitamins, minerals, and antioxidants, supporting immune function and overall health.
- Olive oil adds healthy fats and may help reduce inflammation and improve heart health.
- Low in sodium, suitable for a renal diet.

Preparation Time: 20 minutes

Renal Diet Dinner Recipes for Seniors

1: Baked Lemon Herb Chicken

Ingredients:

- 2 boneless, skinless chicken breasts
- 1 lemon
- 2 cloves garlic, minced

- 1 tablespoon chopped fresh rosemary
- 1 tablespoon chopped fresh thyme
- 1 tablespoon olive oil
- Salt and pepper to taste

Instructions:

- Preheat the oven to 375°F (190°C).
- Place the chicken breasts in a baking dish.
- In a small bowl, combine the juice and zest of the lemon, minced garlic, chopped fresh rosemary, chopped fresh thyme, olive oil, salt, and pepper.
- Pour the lemon herb mixture over the chicken breasts, ensuring they are evenly coated.
- Cover the baking dish with foil and bake in the preheated oven for 25-30 minutes, or until the chicken is cooked through and no longer pink in the center.
- Remove the foil during the last 5 minutes of cooking to allow the chicken to brown slightly.
- Serve hot with steamed vegetables or a side salad.

Health Benefits:

- Chicken breast is a lean source of protein, supporting muscle strength and repair.
- Lemon juice and zest provide vitamin C and antioxidants, boosting immune function and aiding in digestion.
- Fresh herbs like rosemary and thyme add flavor without extra sodium, promoting heart health and reducing inflammation.
- Olive oil provides healthy fats, promoting heart health and reducing the risk of chronic diseases.

Preparation Time: 35 minutes

2: Salmon and Asparagus Foil Packets

Ingredients:

- 2 salmon fillets (4-6 ounces each)
- 1 bunch asparagus, trimmed
- 2 tablespoons olive oil
- 2 cloves garlic, minced
- 1 lemon, thinly sliced
- Salt and pepper to taste

Instructions:

- Preheat the oven to 400°F (200°C).
- Tear off two large pieces of aluminum foil.
- Place each salmon fillet in the center of a piece of foil.
- Arrange the trimmed asparagus around the salmon fillets.
- In a small bowl, combine the olive oil, minced garlic, salt, and pepper.
- Drizzle the olive oil mixture over the salmon and asparagus.
- Place lemon slices on top of the salmon fillets.
- Fold the edges of the foil over the salmon and asparagus to create a sealed packet.
- Place the foil packets on a baking sheet and bake in the preheated oven for 15-20 minutes, or until the salmon is cooked through and flakes easily with a fork.
- Carefully open the foil packets and serve hot.

Health Benefits:

- Salmon is rich in omega-3 fatty acids, which support heart health and reduce inflammation.
- Asparagus is low in potassium and phosphorus, making it kidney-friendly, and provides fiber, vitamins, and antioxidants.
- Garlic adds flavor and has anti-inflammatory and antibacterial properties.
- Lemon slices provide vitamin C and antioxidants, aiding in digestion and immune function.

Preparation Time: 25 minutes

3: Turkey and Vegetable Stir-Fry

Ingredients:

- 4 ounces lean ground turkey
- 1 cup mixed vegetables (such as bell peppers, broccoli, carrots, snap peas)
- 1 tablespoon low-sodium soy sauce
- 1 tablespoon olive oil
- 1 clove garlic, minced
- 1 teaspoon grated ginger

- Salt and pepper to taste
- Cooked brown rice for serving (optional)

Instructions:

- Heat olive oil in a large skillet or wok over medium-high heat.
- Add lean ground turkey to the skillet and cook until browned and cooked through, breaking it into small pieces with a spatula.
- Remove the cooked turkey from the skillet and set aside.
- In the same skillet, add minced garlic and grated ginger, and cook for 1-2 minutes until fragrant.
- Add mixed vegetables to the skillet and stir-fry for 5-7 minutes until tender-crisp.
- Return the cooked turkey to the skillet and stir to combine with the vegetables.
- Drizzle low-sodium soy sauce over the turkey and vegetables, and toss to coat evenly.
- Season with salt and pepper to taste.
- Serve hot over cooked brown rice, if desired.

Health Benefits:

- Lean ground turkey is a good source of protein and low in saturated fat, supporting muscle strength and overall health.
- Mixed vegetables provide vitamins, minerals, and antioxidants, supporting immune function and heart health.
- Garlic and ginger have anti-inflammatory properties and may help lower blood pressure and cholesterol levels.
- Low-sodium soy sauce adds flavor without increasing sodium intake.

Preparation Time: 20 minutes

4: Lentil and Vegetable Curry

Ingredients:

- 1 cup dried green lentils, rinsed
- 2 cups low-sodium vegetable broth
- 1 onion, diced
- 2 cloves garlic, minced
- 1 tablespoon olive oil

- 1 tablespoon curry powder
- 1 teaspoon ground turmeric
- 1 teaspoon ground cumin
- 1 teaspoon ground coriander
- 1 can (14 ounces) diced tomatoes
- 2 cups mixed vegetables (such as cauliflower, carrots, peas)
- Salt and pepper to taste
- Cooked brown rice for serving (optional)

Instructions:

- Heat olive oil in a large pot over medium heat.
- Add diced onion to the pot and cook for 5-7 minutes until softened.
- Add minced garlic, curry powder, ground turmeric, ground cumin, and ground coriander to the pot, and cook for an additional 1-2 minutes until fragrant.
- Stir in rinsed green lentils, low-sodium vegetable broth, diced tomatoes (with juices), and mixed vegetables.

- Bring the mixture to a boil, then reduce heat to low and simmer, covered, for 20-25 minutes until lentils are tender and vegetables are cooked through.
- Season with salt and pepper to taste.
- Serve hot over cooked brown rice, if desired.

Health Benefits:

- Green lentils are a good source of protein and fiber, aiding in satiety and digestive health.
- Mixed vegetables provide vitamins, minerals, and antioxidants, supporting immune function and overall health.
- Curry spices like turmeric, cumin, and coriander have anti-inflammatory properties and may help reduce the risk of chronic diseases.
- Low in sodium and saturated fat, suitable for a renal diet.

Preparation Time: 30 minutes

5: Grilled Lemon Garlic Shrimp Skewers

Ingredients:

- 12 large shrimp, peeled and deveined

- 1 lemon, juiced and zested
- 2 cloves garlic, minced
- 1 tablespoon olive oil
- Salt and pepper to taste
- Optional: Cherry tomatoes, bell peppers, onions (for skewering)

Instructions:

- In a bowl, combine the lemon juice, lemon zest, minced garlic, olive oil, salt, and pepper.
- Add the shrimp to the marinade and toss until evenly coated. Let it marinate for at least 15 minutes.
- Preheat the grill to medium-high heat.
- Thread the marinated shrimp onto skewers, alternating with optional vegetables if desired.
- Grill the skewers for 2-3 minutes on each side, or until the shrimp are pink and opaque.
- Serve hot with a side of steamed vegetables or a green salad.

Health Benefits:

- Shrimp is a low-fat source of protein, supporting muscle strength and repair.
- Lemon juice provides vitamin C and antioxidants, aiding in digestion and boosting immune function.
- Garlic has anti-inflammatory properties and may help lower cholesterol levels and blood pressure.
- Olive oil adds healthy fats and may reduce the risk of heart disease.

Preparation Time: 25 minutes (including marinating time)

6: Baked Herb-Crusted Cod

Ingredients:

- 2 cod fillets (4-6 ounces each)
- 1/4 cup breadcrumbs (whole wheat or gluten-free)
- 1 tablespoon chopped fresh parsley
- 1 tablespoon chopped fresh dill
- 1 tablespoon olive oil
- 1 lemon, sliced
- Salt and pepper to taste

Instructions:

- Preheat the oven to 400°F (200°C).
- In a small bowl, combine the breadcrumbs, chopped fresh parsley, chopped fresh dill, olive oil, salt, and pepper.
- Place the cod fillets on a baking sheet lined with parchment paper.
- Press the breadcrumb mixture onto the top of each cod fillet, coating evenly.
- Place lemon slices on top of the breadcrumb mixture.
- Bake in the preheated oven for 12-15 minutes, or until the fish flakes easily with a fork.
- Serve hot with a side of roasted vegetables or quinoa.

Health Benefits:

- Cod is a lean source of protein and low in saturated fat, supporting muscle health and heart health.
- Fresh herbs like parsley and dill add flavor without extra calories or sodium, and may have anti-inflammatory properties.

- Whole wheat breadcrumbs provide fiber and complex carbohydrates, promoting digestive health and stable blood sugar levels.
- Olive oil adds healthy fats and may reduce inflammation and improve heart health.

Preparation Time: 20 minutes

7: Vegetable and Bean Chili

Ingredients:

- 1 tablespoon olive oil
- 1 onion, diced
- 2 cloves garlic, minced
- 1 bell pepper, diced
- 1 zucchini, diced
- 1 carrot, diced
- 1 can (14 ounces) low-sodium diced tomatoes
- 1 can (14 ounces) low-sodium kidney beans, drained and rinsed
- 1 can (14 ounces) low-sodium black beans, drained and rinsed
- 2 cups low-sodium vegetable broth
- 2 teaspoons chili powder

- 1 teaspoon ground cumin
- Salt and pepper to taste
- Optional toppings: chopped cilantro, diced avocado, Greek yogurt

Instructions:

- Heat olive oil in a large pot over medium heat.
- Add diced onion and minced garlic to the pot and cook for 5-7 minutes until softened.
- Add diced bell pepper, zucchini, and carrot to the pot and cook for an additional 5 minutes.
- Stir in low-sodium diced tomatoes, kidney beans, black beans, vegetable broth, chili powder, ground cumin, salt, and pepper.
- Bring the chili to a boil, then reduce heat to low and simmer, covered, for 20-25 minutes, stirring occasionally.
- Adjust seasoning with additional salt and pepper if needed.
- Serve hot with optional toppings like chopped cilantro, diced avocado, or a dollop of Greek yogurt.

Health Benefits:

- Beans provide plant-based protein and fiber, promoting satiety and digestive health.
- Vegetables add vitamins, minerals, and antioxidants, supporting immune function and overall health.
- Chili powder and cumin add flavor without extra calories or sodium.
- Low-sodium ingredients help maintain kidney health.

Preparation Time: 35 minutes

8: Lemon Herb Baked Chicken Thighs

Ingredients:

- 4 bone-in, skinless chicken thighs
- 1 lemon, juiced and zested
- 2 cloves garlic, minced
- 1 tablespoon chopped fresh rosemary
- 1 tablespoon chopped fresh thyme
- 1 tablespoon olive oil
- Salt and pepper to taste

Instructions:

- Preheat the oven to 375°F (190°C).
- Place the chicken thighs in a baking dish.
- In a small bowl, combine the lemon juice, lemon zest, minced garlic, chopped fresh rosemary, chopped fresh thyme, olive oil, salt, and pepper.
- Pour the lemon herb mixture over the chicken thighs, ensuring they are evenly coated.
- Bake in the preheated oven for 30-35 minutes, or until the chicken is cooked through and juices run clear.
- Serve hot with a side of steamed vegetables or a green salad.

Health Benefits:

- Chicken thighs are a good source of protein and essential nutrients, supporting muscle strength and repair.
- Lemon juice provides vitamin C and antioxidants, aiding in digestion and boosting immune function.

- Fresh herbs like rosemary and thyme add flavor without extra calories or sodium, and may have anti-inflammatory properties.
- Olive oil adds healthy fats and may reduce inflammation and improve heart health.

Preparation Time: 40 minutes

9: Baked Salmon with Roasted Vegetables

Ingredients:

- 2 salmon fillets (4-6 ounces each)
- 1 tablespoon olive oil
- 1 teaspoon dried Italian seasoning
- Salt and pepper to taste
- 1 cup mixed vegetables (such as bell peppers, zucchini, cherry tomatoes)
- 1 tablespoon balsamic vinegar
- Fresh parsley for garnish

Instructions:

- Preheat the oven to 400°F (200°C).
- Place the salmon fillets on a baking sheet lined with parchment paper.

- Drizzle olive oil over the salmon fillets and sprinkle with dried Italian seasoning, salt, and pepper.
- In a separate bowl, toss the mixed vegetables with olive oil, balsamic vinegar, salt, and pepper.
- Arrange the mixed vegetables around the salmon fillets on the baking sheet.
- Bake in the preheated oven for 12-15 minutes, or until the salmon is cooked through and flakes easily with a fork.
- Garnish with fresh parsley before serving.

Health Benefits:

- Salmon is rich in omega-3 fatty acids, which support heart health and reduce inflammation.
- Mixed vegetables provide vitamins, minerals, and antioxidants, supporting immune function and overall health.
- Olive oil adds healthy fats and may reduce inflammation and improve heart health.
- Balsamic vinegar adds flavor without extra sodium.

Preparation Time: 20 minutes

10: Turkey and Vegetable Skillet

Ingredients:

- 8 ounces lean ground turkey
- 1 tablespoon olive oil
- 1 onion, diced
- 2 cloves garlic, minced
- 1 bell pepper, diced
- 1 zucchini, diced
- 1 cup cherry tomatoes, halved
- 1 teaspoon dried oregano
- Salt and pepper to taste
- Fresh basil for garnish

Instructions:

- Heat olive oil in a large skillet over medium heat.
- Add diced onion and minced garlic to the skillet and cook for 5-7 minutes until softened.
- Add lean ground turkey to the skillet and cook until browned, breaking it into small pieces with a spatula.
- Stir in diced bell pepper, diced zucchini, halved cherry tomatoes, dried oregano, salt, and pepper.

- Cook for an additional 5-7 minutes until the vegetables are tender.
- Garnish with fresh basil before serving.

Health Benefits:

- Lean ground turkey is a good source of protein and low in saturated fat, supporting muscle health and heart health.
- Vegetables provide vitamins, minerals, and antioxidants, supporting immune function and overall health.
- Olive oil adds healthy fats and may reduce inflammation and improve heart health.
- Fresh basil adds flavor without extra calories or sodium.

Preparation Time: 25 minutes

Renal Diet Snacks Recipes for Seniors

1: Greek Yogurt and Berry Parfait

Ingredients:

- 1/2 cup low-fat Greek yogurt

- 1/4 cup mixed berries (such as strawberries, blueberries, raspberries)
- 1 tablespoon chopped nuts (such as almonds, walnuts)
- 1 teaspoon honey or maple syrup (optional)
- Dash of cinnamon (optional)

Instructions:

- In a small bowl or glass, layer the Greek yogurt, mixed berries, and chopped nuts.
- Drizzle with honey or maple syrup if desired.
- Sprinkle with a dash of cinnamon for extra flavor.
- Serve immediately and enjoy!

Health Benefits:

- Greek yogurt is high in protein and calcium, promoting muscle strength and bone health.
- Berries are rich in antioxidants and fiber, supporting immune function and digestive health.
- Nuts provide healthy fats and protein, aiding in satiety and heart health.

- Honey or maple syrup adds natural sweetness without extra sodium.

Preparation Time: 5 minutes

2: Veggie Sticks with Hummus

Ingredients:

- Assorted vegetable sticks (such as carrots, celery, bell peppers, cucumber)
- 1/4 cup hummus (store-bought or homemade)

Instructions:

- Wash and cut assorted vegetables into sticks.
- Arrange the vegetable sticks on a plate or in a container.
- Serve with hummus for dipping.
- Enjoy as a nutritious snack!

Health Benefits:

- Vegetables are low in calories and high in vitamins, minerals, and antioxidants, promoting overall health and reducing the risk of chronic diseases.

- Hummus provides protein and fiber, aiding in satiety and digestive health.
- This snack is low in sodium and suitable for a renal diet, helping to maintain kidney health.

Preparation Time: 10 minutes

3: Cottage Cheese and Fruit Bowl

Ingredients:

- 1/2 cup low-fat cottage cheese
- 1/4 cup mixed fruit (such as pineapple chunks, grapes, kiwi slices)
- 1 tablespoon chopped nuts (such as pecans, pistachios)
- 1 teaspoon honey (optional)

Instructions:

- In a bowl, place the low-fat cottage cheese.
- Top with mixed fruit and chopped nuts.
- Drizzle with honey if desired for added sweetness.
- Mix gently and enjoy!

Health Benefits:

- Cottage cheese is a good source of protein and calcium, promoting muscle strength and bone health.
- Mixed fruits provide vitamins, minerals, and antioxidants, supporting immune function and overall health.
- Nuts add healthy fats and protein, aiding in satiety and heart health.
- Honey adds natural sweetness without extra sodium.

Preparation Time: 5 minutes

4: Avocado and Tomato Toast

Ingredients:

- 1 slice whole grain bread, toasted
- 1/4 ripe avocado, mashed
- 1 small tomato, sliced
- Pinch of salt and pepper
- Optional toppings: sliced radishes, microgreens, balsamic glaze

Instructions:

- Toast the slice of whole grain bread until golden brown.
- Spread the mashed avocado evenly on top of the toast.
- Arrange sliced tomatoes on top of the avocado.
- Season with a pinch of salt and pepper.
- Optionally, garnish with sliced radishes, microgreens, or a drizzle of balsamic glaze.
- Serve immediately and enjoy!

Health Benefits:

- Whole grain bread provides fiber and complex carbohydrates, promoting digestive health and stable blood sugar levels.
- Avocado is rich in healthy fats, vitamins, and minerals, supporting heart health and brain function.
- Tomatoes are high in antioxidants and vitamins, promoting immune function and reducing inflammation.
- This snack is low in sodium and suitable for a renal diet, helping to maintain kidney health.

Preparation Time: 10 minutes

5: Egg Salad Cucumber Bites

Ingredients:

- 2 hard-boiled eggs, peeled and chopped
- 2 tablespoons Greek yogurt
- 1 teaspoon Dijon mustard
- 1 tablespoon chopped chives or green onions
- Salt and pepper to taste
- 1 cucumber, sliced into rounds

Instructions:

- In a bowl, mix together the chopped hard-boiled eggs, Greek yogurt, Dijon mustard, chopped chives or green onions, salt, and pepper until well combined.
- Place cucumber slices on a serving plate.
- Spoon a small amount of the egg salad mixture onto each cucumber slice.
- Garnish with additional chopped chives or green onions if desired.
- Serve immediately and enjoy!

Health Benefits:

- Hard-boiled eggs provide protein and essential nutrients, supporting muscle strength and overall health.
- Greek yogurt adds creaminess and protein to the egg salad, aiding in muscle repair and promoting satiety.
- Cucumber slices are low in calories and high in water content, helping to stay hydrated and promoting healthy skin.
- This snack is low in sodium and suitable for a renal diet, helping to maintain kidney health.

Preparation Time: 15 minutes

6: Almond Butter Apple Slices

Ingredients:

- 1 medium apple, sliced
- 2 tablespoons almond butter
- 1 tablespoon unsweetened shredded coconut
- 1 tablespoon chopped almonds

Instructions:

- Slice the apple into thin rounds or wedges, removing the core.
- Spread almond butter on each apple slice.
- Sprinkle unsweetened shredded coconut and chopped almonds over the almond butter.
- Serve immediately and enjoy!

Health Benefits:

- Apples are rich in fiber and antioxidants, promoting digestive health and reducing the risk of chronic diseases.
- Almond butter provides healthy fats, protein, and fiber, aiding in satiety and heart health.
- Shredded coconut and chopped almonds add texture and additional nutrients, such as healthy fats and vitamins.
- This snack is low in sodium and suitable for a renal diet, helping to maintain kidney health.

Preparation Time: 5 minutes

7: Tuna and Cucumber Roll-Ups

Ingredients:

- 1 can (5 ounces) tuna, drained
- 2 tablespoons Greek yogurt
- 1 tablespoon chopped fresh dill or parsley
- Salt and pepper to taste
- 1 cucumber, peeled into thin strips using a vegetable peeler

Instructions:

- In a bowl, mix together the drained tuna, Greek yogurt, chopped fresh dill or parsley, salt, and pepper until well combined.
- Lay a cucumber strip flat on a clean surface.
- Spoon a small amount of the tuna mixture onto one end of the cucumber strip.
- Roll up the cucumber strip tightly, enclosing the tuna mixture.
- Secure with a toothpick if needed.
- Repeat with the remaining cucumber strips and tuna mixture.
- Serve immediately or refrigerate until ready to eat.

Health Benefits:

- Tuna is a lean source of protein and omega-3 fatty acids, supporting muscle strength and heart health.
- Greek yogurt adds creaminess and protein to the tuna mixture, aiding in muscle repair and promoting satiety.
- Cucumber is low in calories and high in water content, helping to stay hydrated and promoting healthy skin.
- This snack is low in sodium and suitable for a renal diet, helping to maintain kidney health.

Preparation Time: 10 minutes

8: Rice Cake with Avocado and Tomato

Ingredients:

- 1 rice cake
- 1/4 ripe avocado, mashed
- 1 small tomato, sliced
- Salt and pepper to taste
- Optional toppings: sliced radishes, microgreens, balsamic glaze

Instructions:

- Spread the mashed avocado evenly on top of the rice cake.
- Arrange sliced tomatoes on top of the avocado.
- Season with a pinch of salt and pepper.
- Optionally, garnish with sliced radishes, microgreens, or a drizzle of balsamic glaze.
- Serve immediately and enjoy!

Health Benefits:

- Rice cakes are low in calories and provide complex carbohydrates for energy.
- Avocado is rich in healthy fats, vitamins, and minerals, supporting heart health and brain function.
- Tomatoes are high in antioxidants and vitamins, promoting immune function and reducing inflammation.
- This snack is low in sodium and suitable for a renal diet, helping to maintain kidney health.

Preparation Time: 5 minutes

9: Hummus-Stuffed Mini Bell Peppers

Ingredients:

- 6 mini bell peppers
- 1/2 cup hummus (store-bought or homemade)
- Optional toppings: chopped fresh parsley, paprika, sesame seeds

Instructions:

- Slice each mini bell pepper in half lengthwise and remove the seeds.
- Fill each pepper half with a spoonful of hummus.
- Optionally, sprinkle chopped fresh parsley, paprika, or sesame seeds on top for added flavor and presentation.
- Arrange the stuffed bell peppers on a serving plate.
- Serve immediately or refrigerate until ready to eat.

Health Benefits:

- Bell peppers are low in potassium and rich in vitamins A and C, promoting eye health and immune function.

- Hummus provides plant-based protein and fiber, aiding in satiety and digestive health.
- This snack is low in sodium and suitable for a renal diet, helping to maintain kidney health.

Preparation Time: 10 minutes

10: Cottage Cheese and Tomato Slices

Ingredients:

- 1/2 cup low-fat cottage cheese
- 1 small tomato, sliced
- Fresh basil leaves for garnish
- Balsamic glaze for drizzling (optional)

Instructions:

- Arrange the tomato slices on a serving plate.
- Spoon low-fat cottage cheese onto each tomato slice.
- Garnish with fresh basil leaves.
- Optionally, drizzle with balsamic glaze for added flavor.
- Serve immediately and enjoy!

Health Benefits:

- Cottage cheese is a good source of protein and calcium, supporting muscle strength and bone health.
- Tomatoes are rich in antioxidants and vitamins, promoting immune function and reducing inflammation.
- Fresh basil adds flavor and may have anti-inflammatory properties.
- This snack is low in sodium and suitable for a renal diet, helping to maintain kidney health.

Preparation Time: 5 minutes

CONCLUSION

The Renal Diet Cookbook for Seniors offers a comprehensive guide to promoting kidney health while enjoying delicious and nourishing meals.

By emphasizing nutrient-rich ingredients, thoughtful recipes, and mindful portion sizes, this cookbook empowers seniors to take control of their dietary choices and optimize their well-being.

Through a variety of breakfast, lunch, dinner, and snack options, seniors can discover flavorful dishes that align with their renal diet requirements without sacrificing taste or satisfaction.

From vibrant salads to hearty soups, each recipe is carefully crafted to support kidney function, manage nutrient intake, and enhance overall health.

This cookbook goes beyond mere recipes, providing valuable insights into the principles of renal nutrition and practical tips for meal planning, grocery shopping, and dining out.

With accessible ingredients and easy-to-follow instructions, seniors can confidently navigate their dietary needs and embark on a journey toward better health and vitality.

The Renal Diet Cookbook for Seniors serves as a trusted companion on the path to improved kidney function and enhanced quality of life.

Whether you're a senior managing kidney disease or simply seeking to adopt a kidney-friendly lifestyle, this cookbook offers a wealth of resources and inspiration for nourishing your body, mind, and spirit.

www.ingramcontent.com/pod-product-compliance
Lightning Source LLC
Chambersburg PA
CBHW070354230526
45471CB00006B/2557